The Ultimate Guide To:

<u>Appetizers</u>

Yummy & Delicious Appetizer Recipes That Are Mouthwatering, Healthy & Easy To Make For Beginners

Table Of Contents

Introduction

Chapter 1: Best Appetizer Recipes 1

Chapter 2: Best Appetizer Recipes 2

Chapter 3: Best Appetizer Recipes 3

Chapter 4: Best Appetizer Recipes 4

Chapter 5: Delicious Recipes 1

Chapter 6: Delicious Recipes 2

Chapter 7: Delicious Recipes 3

Chapter 8: Delicious Recipe 4

Conclusion

Disclaimer Notice

Introduction

Appetizers can often be the best part of a meal and many people prefer them to larger courses. Indeed they are so popular that sometimes whole dinner parties consist entirely of a variety of appetizers, or for those dining out, the temptations is often to order a variety of appetizers instead of a main course.

You can see the attraction –appetizers by definition indicate small portions, which mean there could be a wide and delicious selection of different and interesting dishes from which diners can pick and choose. Of course, for the cook, having to provide such a medley of diverse foods can be quite a challenge (although one may well fell equal to), but for the guests it will be nothing less than a complete delight. They are ideal for getting any meal or party off to the best possible start.

The deliciously tempting recipes in this book are clearly explained in steps making it ideal for the first time cook as well as the more experienced one, who will find lots of tempting dishes suited In some countries, appetizers, or starters, have become an institution. Italian antipasto is so varied and delicious that you'd be forgiven for wishing to stop right there with the artichokes and superb dried hams, and forget entirely about the pasta and meat the follow.

Where you want appetizers to start off a meal or to serve as a buffet spread, this collection of delicious recipes will fit the bill. Here in one volume is an incredible choice of delectable little morsels to whet the appetite and leave the diner ready for more. This unique book has combined recipes from all over the world to assist you in creating various types of appetizers that everyone will enjoy no matter the occasion.

With the wealth of idea, you will be spoilt for choice. There are classics such as French Onion soup or Roasted tomatoes and Mozzarella with basil oil; Mediterranean favorites such as Tapenade and Aioli with vegetables; Scallops wrapped in prosciutto for a stylish dinner; tasty party bites such as mini saffron fish cakes and fiery tuna spring rolls; and more substantial snacks and first courses such as beef empanadas or halloumi and grape salad

Thank you for purchasing this book and I wish you good luck!

Chapter 1: Best Appetizer Recipes 1

Recipe #1; Fiery Guacamole

One of the best loves Mexican salsas, this blend of creamy avocados, tomatoes, chilies, coriander and lime now appears on tables the world over. Bought guacamole usually contains mayonnaise, which helps to preserve the avocado, but this is not an ingredient in traditional recipes. Serves 6-8

Ingredients

4 medium tomatoes

4 ripe avocados, preferably fuerte

Juice of 1 lime

Half small onion

2 garlic cloves

Small bunch of fresh coriander chopped

3 fresh red fresh chillies

Salt

Tortilla chips to serve

1. Cut across into the base of each tomato. Place the tomatoes in a heat proof bowl and pour over boiling water to cover
2. Leave the tomatoes in the water for 3 minutes, then lift them out using a slotted spoon and plung them into a bowl of cold water. Drain. The skins will have

begun to peel back from the crosses

3. Cut the avocados in half, then remove the stones(pits). Scoop the flesh out of the shells and put in a food processor or blender. Process until almost smooth, then scrape into a bowl then stirs the lime juice.
4. Chop the onions finely then crush the garlic. Add both to the avocado and mix well. Stir the coriander.
5. Remove the stalks from the chillies, slit them and scrape out the seeds with a small sharp knife. Chop the chillies finely and add them to the avocado mixture with the chopped tomatoes. Mix well.
6. Check the seasoning and add salt to taste. Cover closely with clear film (plastic wrap) or a tight fitting lid and chill for one hour before serving as a deep with tortilla chips. If it is well covered guacamole will keep in the refrigerator for 2-3 days.

Recipe #2; Tapenade with Quail's Eggs and Crudites

This tasty olive based spread or dip makes a social able start to a meal for friends.

Ingredients

2 cups pitted black olives

2 large garlic cloves peeled

1 tbsp salted capers, rinsed

6 canned or bottled anchovy fillets, drained

50g good quality canned tuna

10ml cognac (optional)

1 tbsp chopped thyme

2 tbsp chopped fresh parsley

4 tbsp extra virgin olive oil

A dash of lemon juice

2 tbsp crème fraiche or framage frais (optional)

12-18 quails eggs

Ground black pepper

For the crudités

Bunch of spring onions (scallions) halved if large

Bunch of radishes, trimmed and halved if large, or 1 large fennel bulb, cut into thin wedges

To serve

French bread

Unsalted (sweet) butter or olive oil and sea salt to dip

1. Process the olives, garlic cloves, capers, anchovies and tuna in a food processor or blender. Transfer into a mixing bowl and stir in the cognac, if using the thyme, parsley and enough olive oil to make the paste. Season to taste with pepper and a dash of lemon juice. Stir in the crème fraiche or fromage frais, if using and transfer to a serving bowl.
2. Place the quail's eggs in a pan of cold water and bring to the boil. Cook for 2 minutes only, then immediately drain and plunge the eggs into iced water to stop them

from cooking any further and to help make them easier to shell. When the eggs are cold, carefully part shell them.

3. Serve the tapenade with the eggs and crudités and offer chunks of crusty French bread, unsalted or olive oil and sea salt alongside.

Recipe #3; Taramasalata

This delicious specialty makes an excellent start to any meal, accompanied by fruity black olives and slices of warm pitta bread. This is one of the most famous Greek dips, and central part of nay meze table, home-made taramasalata is incomparably better than the readymade versions sold in supermarkets. Serves 4

Ingredients

4oz smoked mullet roe or smoked cods roe

2 garlic cloves, crushed

2 tbsp grated onions

4 tbsp olive oil

4 slices white bread crusts removed

Juice of 2 lemons

2 tbsp milk or water

Ground black pepper

Warm pitta bread to serve

1. Place the smoked fish roe, garlic, grated onions, oil,

bread and lemon juice in a blender or food processor until the mixtures is smooth

2. Scrape down the edges of the food processor or blender to ensure that all the ingredients are properly incorporated. Blend quickly again.

3. Add the milk or water and process again for few seconds. (this will give the taramasalata a creamier texture)

4. Pour the taramasalata into a serving bowl, cover with clear film (plastic wrap) and chill for 1-2 hours before serving. Sprinkle the dip with black pepper and serve with warm pitta bread

Cook's tips

The smoked roe of grey millet is traditionally used for rtaramasalata, but it is expensive and can be difficult to obtain. Smoked cod roe is often used instead to make this dish. It varies in color and may be paler than the burnt orange color of mullet roe, nut it still very good. When buying smoked cod's roe, make sure that it is not overcooked as this makes it hard and prevents it blending well.

Recipe #4; Brandade of salt Cod

There are many versions of this creamy French salt cod puree. Some contain mashed potatoes, others truffles. Serve the brandade with warmed crisbread or crusty bread for tasty appetizers, or for a light lunch. Serve the brandade and bread with tomato and basil salad. You can omit the garlic from the brandade. If you prefer, and serve toasted slices of crusty French bread rubbed with garlic instead. Serves 6

Ingredients

200g salt cod

250ml cup of extra virgin oil

4 garlic cloves, crushed

250ml double (heavy) or whipping cream

1. Soak the salt cod in a bowl of cold water for 24 hours changing the water frequently
2. Drain the fish well, cut the fish into pieces, place in a shallow pan and pour in enough cold water to cover. Heat the water until is simmering and poach the fish for 8 minutes, until it is just cooked
3. Drain the fish thoroughly, then carefully remove the skin and bones with a sharp knife
4. Combine the extra virgin oil and crushed garlic cloves in a small pan and heat gently
5. In another pan heat the double cream or whipping cream until it starts to simmer
6. Put the cod into a food processor, process it briefly, then gradually add alternative amounts of the garlic flavored olive oil and cream. While continuing to process the mixture. The aim is to create a puree with the consistency of mashed potato.
7. Season to taste with ground black pepper, then scoop the brandade into a serving or on to individual serving plates and serve with crisp bread or crusty bread.

Recipe #5; Thousand Island Dip

This variation on the classic Thousand Island dressing is far removed from the original version, but can be served in the same way. With shellfish lace on to bamboo skewers for dipping or with a simple salad as a tasty appetizer. Serves 4

Ingredients

4 sun dried tomatoes in oil

4 plum tomatoes or 2 beefsteak tomatoes

150g mild soft cheese or mascarpone or framage frais

4 tbsp mayonnaise

2 tbsp tomato purees (paste)

2 tbsp chopped fresh parsley

1 lemon

Tobacco sauce to taste

1 tbsp Worcestershire sauce or soy sauce

Salt and ground pepper

1. Drain the oil from the sun dried tomatoes then cut them into small pieces
2. Cut a cross in the blossom end of each fresh tomato, place them in a heat proof bowl and pour over boiling water. Leave for 1-2 minutes, then lift them out and peel of the skin
3. Chop the flesh finely, put the sun dried tomatoes and fresh chopped tomatoes in separate bowls and set them aside
4. Put the soft cheese in a bowl. Beat it until it is creamy, then gradually beat in the mayonnaise. Add the tomatoes puree in the same way.
5. Stir in the parsley and sun dried tomatoes, the fresh sliced tomatoes. Mix well until the mixture is evenly colored.
6. Grate the lemon finely and add the grinds in the dip. Mix well squeeze the lemon and add the juice into the

bowl, with tobacco sauce to taste. Stir in the Worcestershire sauce or soy sauce and salt and black ground pepper to taste.

7. Spoon the dip into a serving bowl, swirling the surface attractively. Cover with clear film (plastic wrap) and chill in the refrigerator until ready to serve.

Chapter 2: Best Appetizer Recipes 2

Recipe #6; Salmon Dip

This creamy salmon dip can be served as an appetizer or part of the buffet lunch. Serves 4

Ingredients

115g smoked salmon diced

250g mascarpone cheese

Grated ring and juice of one lemon

1 red bell (pepper), seeded and cut into strips

One yellow bell pepper, seeded and cut into strips

Sea salt and black ground pepper

For the potato wedges

675g potatoes, scrubbed

4 tbsp olive oil

2 tbsp fresh chopped rose mary

1 fresh red chilli, seeded and finely chopped

1. Preheat the oven into 200c. To make the potato wedges, cut the potatoes into thick wedges. Pour he oil into a roasting pan and heat in the oven for 10 minutes. Add the potato wedges on the hot pan and

sprinkle over with rosemary and chilli.

2. Coat the potato wedges in the oil with rose mary and chilli. Season well with salt and black pepper. Bake for 50-60 minutes or until tender, turning alternatively to prevent the wedges from sticking to the roasting pan

3. Put the mascarpone cheese, chive and lemon rind into a bowl and mix with fork until thoroughly blended

4. Add the lemon juice into the cheese mixture, a little at a time, mixing constantly, so that the mixture is thinned and given a lemony tangy but does not curdle. A reamer (a ridged, tear shaped tool) is useful for squeezing the lemon but watch out for any pips (seeds) that might fall into the bowl.

5. Add the salmon pieces into the cheese mixture and season with ground black pepper to taste. Transfer into a serving bowl and let chill until it ready to serve

6. To serve arrange the pepper strips and potato wedges around the edge of the serving platter and place the dip to one side or in the centre

Recipe #7; Feta and roast Pepper Dip with Chillies

This is a familiar meze in northern Greece, where it is eaten as a dip with pitas, with other dishes, or with toast to accompany a glass of ouzo. The strong, salty feta cheese with the smoky peppers and hot chillies makes a powerful combination to enliven the taste buds. In Greek it is known as htipiyi, which literally means that which is beaten. Serves 4

Ingredients

1 yellow or green bell pepper

1-2 fresh green chillies

200g feta cheese

4 tbsp extra virgin olive oil

Juice of 1 lemon

4 tbsp milk

Ground black pepper

A little finely chopped fresh flat leaf parsley, to garnish slices of toasted Greek bread or pitas, to serve

1. Thread the pepper and the chillies on a metal skewers and turn them over a flame or under the grill(broiler) until the skins are charred all over
2. Put the pepper and the chillies in a plastic bag or in a covered bowl and set them aside until cool enough to handle.
3. Peel off the much of the pepper and chilli skins as possible and wipe the blackened bits off with kitchen paper. Slit the pepper and chillies and discard the seeds and stems.
4. Put the peppers and chillies flesh into a food processor. Add all the other ingredients except the parsley and blend to fairly smooth paste. Add a little more milk if the mixture seems too stiff. Spread on slices of toast, sprinkle a hint of parsley on top and serve.

Variations

Add 75g sun dried tomatoes bottled in oil, drained, to the mixture in the food processor.

Recipe #8; Blue Cheese Dip

This rich delectable dip can be mixed up in next to no time and is delicious. Served with pears, or with fresh vegetables crudités as an appetizer. Add extra yogurt to make a great dressing for a mixed salad. Serves 4

Ingredients

150g blue cheese, such as stilton or Danish blue

150g soft cheese

5 tbsp Greek (US strained yogurt)

Salt and ground pepper

1. Crumble the blue cheese into a bowl, using a wooden spoon, beat the cheese to soften it.
2. Add the soft cheese and beat well until the two chesses are blended together
3. Gradually beat the Greek style yogurt into the bowl of blended cheese, adding enough to give you the constituency you prefer.
4. Season with lots of ground black pepper. Cover and chill the dip in the refrigerator until you are ready to serve

Cook's Tips

The thinner version of this dip is made by adding a little more yogurt and is the classic accompaniment to Buffalo wings. This deep fried chicken wings are names after the city of Buffalo in the states of New York in the USA. There they will invariably come with a bowl of blue cheese dressing on the side for dipping the wings.

Variations

This a very thick dip to which you can add a little more of

Greek style yogurt, or stir in a little milk, for a softer and thinner constituency, if you prefer.

Recipe #9; Bread Sticks

This crispy bread sticks make a tasty snack or appetizer alongside a dip. Serves 8-10

Ingredients

1 **t**bsp active dried yeast

300ml Luke warm water

425g strong white bread flour

2 tbsp salt

1 tbsp Custer (superfine) sugar

2 tbsp olive oil

1 beaten egg for glazing

Coarse salt, for sprinkling

1. Combine the yeast and water, stir and leave for 25 minutes to dissolve
2. Place the flour, salt, sugar and olive oil in a food processor. With the motor running, slowly pour in the yeast mixture, and process until the dough forms a ball. If sticky, add more flour, if dry add more water.
3. Transfer to a floured surface and knead until smooth. Place in a bowl, cover and leave to rise in a warm place for 45 minutes.
4. Lightly toast the sesame seeds in a frying pan. Grease two baking sheets

5. Roll small handfuls of dough into cylinders, about 30cm long. Place on the baking sheets. Brush with egg glaze, sprinkle the sesame seeds, then sprinkle over some coarse salt. Leave to rise, uncovered, until almost doubled in volume about 20 minutes.
6. Preheat the oven to 200c. bake the bread sticks until golden brown about 15 minutes. Turn off the heat but leave the bread sticks in the oven for 5 minutes more. Serve warm or leave to cool before serving.

Recipe #10; Prosciutto and Mozzarella Parcels

Italian prosciutto crudo is a delicious raw smoked ham. Here it is baked with melting mozzarella in a pastry case. Serves 6

Ingredients

A little hot chilli sauce

6 prosciutto slices

200g mozzarella cheese, cut into 6 slices

6 sheets for pastry, each measuring 45 by 28cm

Thawed if frozen

50g butter melted

150g frisee lettuce to serve

1. Preheat the oven to 200c. Sprinkle a little chilli sauce over the prosciutto. Top with a slice of mozzarella, and then fold it around the cheese so the cheese is enclosed by the ham.
2. Brush a sheet of foil pastry with melted butter and fold it in half. Place a ham and mozzarella parcel in

the middle the pastry. Brush the remaining pastry with butter, and then fold it to make a neat parcel. Repeat with the remaining parcels and sheets.

3. Brush all the parcels with butter. Bake for 15 minutes, until the pastry is golden. Serve immediately.

Chapter 3: Best Appetizer Recipes 3

Recipe #11; Navajo Fried Bread

These bread rounds are well served with salsa. Serves 4

Ingredients

2 cups plain all purpose flour

2 tbsp baking powder

2 tbsp salt

1 cup of Luke warm water

Oil for frying

1. Sift the flour, baking powder and salt into a bowl. Pour in the lukewarm water and stir quickly with a fork until the dough gathers into a ball
2. With floured hands, gently knead the dough by rolling it around the bowl. Be careful not to over knead, the dough should be very soft
3. Divide the dough into 8 pieces. With floured hands, pat each piece into a roundabout 13cm in diameter. Place the rounds on a floured baking sheet.
4. Put a 2.5cm layer of oil in a heavy frying pan and heat until hot but not smoking. To taste the temperature, drop in a small piece of the dough, if the oil bubbles immediately then it's ready.
5. Add the dough rounds into the hot oil and press down with a slotted spoon to submerge them. Release the dough and cook until puffed and golden brown on both sides. 3 – 4 minutes turning for even browning.

Fry in batches if necessary.

6. Drain the bread on kitchen paper and serve immediately. They are good to accompaniment to a spicy chilli or with grated cheese and an assortment of homemade salsa and guacamole

Cook's Tip

This fried bread are best eaten on the day they are made because they are not good for keeps.

Recipe #12; Monte Cristo Triangles

These opulent little sandwiches are stuffed with ham, cheese and turkey, dipped in egg, than fried in butter and oil. They are rich and filling. Serves 8

Ingredients

16 thin slices firm textured white bread

120g butter, softened

8 slices oak smoked ham

Whole gram mustard

8 slices gruyere or emmenthal cheese

3-4 tbsp mayonnaise

8 slices cooked turkey or chicken breast fillets

4-5 eggs

50ml milk

5ml dijan mustard

Vegetable oil, for frying

Butter for frying

For Garnish

Pimiento-stuffed green olives fresh parsley leaves

1. Arrange eight of the bread slices on a work surface and spread with half the softened butter. Lay a slice of ham on each piece of bread and spread with a little mustard. Cover with a slice of gruyere or emmenthal cheese and spread with a little of the mayonnaise, then cover with a slice of turkey or chicken. Butter the rest of the bread slices and use to top the sandwiches. Cut the crusts, trimming to an even square.
2. In a large shallow oven proof dish, beat the eggs with the milk and Dijon mustard until thoroughly combined. Season to taste with salt and pepper. Soak the sandwich in the egg mixture on both sides until all the has been absorbed.
3. Heat about 1cm of oil with little butter in a large heavy frying pan, until hot, but not smoking. Gently fry the sandwich, in batches for about 4-5 minutes until crisp and golden, turning once. Add more oil and butter as necessary. Drain on kitchen paper.
4. Transfer the sandwich to a chopping board and cut each into four triangles, then cut each in half again. Make 64 triangles in total. Thread an olive oil and parsley leaf on to a cocktail stick (toothpick), then stick into each triangle and serve while warm.

Recipe #13; Homemade Crisp Rye Breads

These traditional crisp breads are from Sweden and were

originally made with a hole in the centre so they could be hung over the oven to keep dry. Nowadays, they keep well in an alright container. They are ideal as a snack or appetizer spread with pate or soft cheese. Makes 15

Ingredients

600ml milk

50g fresh yeast

5 cups rye flour plus

2 cups for dusting

5 cups strong white bread flour

2 tbsp caraway or cumin seeds

1 tbsp salt

1. Put the milk in a pan and heat gently warm to the touch. Remove from the heat. In a bowl, blend the yeast with a little of the warmed milk. Add the remaining milk, then add the rye flour, bread flour, caraway or cumin seeds and salt and mix together to form a dough
2. Using the rye flour for dusting, turn the dough out on to a lightly floured surface and knead the dough for about 2 minutes. Cut the dough into 15 equal pieces, then roll out each piece into a thin, flat round. Place on baking sheets and leave to rise in a warm place for 20 minutes
3. Preheat the oven to 150c. using the rye flour, roll out the pieces of dough again into very thin, flat rounds. Return to the baking sheets. Make a pattern on the surface using a fork or knife
4. ·

5. Bake the bread in the oven for 8-10 minutes, turning after 5 minutes, until hard and crispy. Transfer to a wire rack and leave to cool. Store the bread in an airtight container

Cook's Tip

The Swedes use a special rolling pin with a knobby surface to create the distinctive texture of this hard bread. An ordinary rolling pin is a good substitute, with the speckled texture created with the head of a fork or a knife end.

Recipe #14; Garlic-infused Spicy Bean Dip

Broad beans also known as fava beans are among the oldest vegetables in cultivation, and are staple ingredients in the cuisines on North Africa, where they are native and are eaten both fresh and dried. This delicious garlic and been dip comes from Morocco. Sprinkled with paprika or dried thyme, it makes a tasty appetizer and is best served with armed flat bread or slices of toasted pitta bread. Serves 4

Ingredients

350g dried broad (fava) beans, soaked overnight

4 garlic cloves

2tbsp cumin seeds

4-5 tbsp olive oil

Salt

Paprika or dried thyme to garnish

1. Drain the beans, remove their wrinkly skins and place them in a large pan with the garlic and cumin seeds.
2. Add enough water to cover the beans and bring to the boil. Boil vigorously for about 10 minutes, skimming off any scum that rises to the surface
3. Reduce the heat, cover the pan and simmer the beans gently for about 1 hour, or until they are tender
4. Drain the beans and while they are still warm, pound them in a mortar and pestle or use a food processor or a blender to process them with olive oil until the mixture forms a smooth dip
5. Season to taste with salt and serve warm or at room temperature, sprinkled with paprika.

Cook's tip

A good ways of saving the energy while cooking the beans is to tightly cover the pan after boiling the beans and then turn off the heat. The beans can be left to cook in the slowly cooling water in the pan for about 3-4 hours, by which time they should be tender.

Recipe #15; Hummus

T his classic chickpea dip from the eastern Mediterranean is a firm favorite everywhere. It is flavored with garlic and tahini-sesame seed paste. For extra flavor, a little ground cumin can be added and olive oil can also be stirred in to enrich the hummus, if you like. It is lovely served with wedges of toasted pitta or with crudités as a delicious dip. Serves 4-6

Ingredients

400g can chickpeas, drained

4 tbsp tahini

3 garlic gloves, chopped

Lemon juice half a cup

Salt and ground black pepper

A few whole chickpeas reserved to garnish

1. Reserving a few for garnish, coarsely mash the chick peas in a mixing bowl with a fork. If you like a smoother puree, process the chickpeas in a food processor or blender until a smooth paste is formed
2. Mix the tahini into a bowl of chickpeas, then stir in the chopped garlic cloves and lemon juice. Season to taste and garnish the top with the reserved chickpeas. Serve the hummus at room temperature.

Variations

Process 2 roasted red (bell) pepper with the chickpeas, then continue as above. Serve sprinkled with lightly toasted pine nuts and paprika mixed with a little extra virgin olive oil. Add a pinch of cayenne to the mixture Instead of chickpeas, top with a drizzle of olive oil and a dusting of paprika

Cook's Tip

Add more lemon juice to taste if necessary when seasoning

Chapter 4: Best Appetizer Recipes 4

Recipe #16; Baba Ganoush with Lebanese Flatbread

Baba Ganoush is a delectable aubergine dip from the Middle East. Tahini-sesame seed paste and ground cumin are the main flavoring, giving a subtle hint of spice. Serves 6

Ingredients

2 small aubergines (eggplants)

1 garlic clove, crushed

4 tbsp tahini

25g ground almonds

A half a cup of lemon juice

A half tbsp of ground cumin

2 tbsp fresh mint leaves

2 tbsp olive oil

1. Start by making the Lebanese flat bread. Split the pitta breads horizontally through the middle and carefully open them out flat, cut side up. Mix the sesame seeds, chopped thyme and poppy seeds in a mortar. Crush the lightly with pestle to release their flavor
2. Stir the olive oil into the spice mixture. Spread the mixture lightly over the cut sides of the pitta bread, grill until golden brown and crisp. When cool enough to handle, break into rough pieces and set aside

3. Grill the aubergines, turning them several times, till the skin is darkened and blistered. Do away with the skin, chop the flesh in chunks and leave to drain in the colander

4. Squeeze out as much liquid from the aubergine as possible. Place the flesh in a blender or food processor. Add the garlic, tahini, ground cumin, almonds and the lemon juice with salt to taste and process to a smooth paste. Roughly chop half the mint and stir into the dip.

5. Spoon into a bowl, sprinkle the remaining leaves on top and drizzle with olive oil. Serve with Lebanese flat bread

Recipe #17; Tsatziki

Cool creamy and refreshing tsatziki is wonderfully easy to make and even easier to eat. Serve this classic Greek dip with toasted pitta bread as part of a salad spread, or with char grilled vegetables. Serves 4

Ingredients

1 mini cucumber, topped and tailed

4 spring onions

1 garlic clove

200ml Greek (US strained plain) yoghurt

1 garlic clove

45ml chopped fresh mint

Salt and ground black pepper

Fresh mint sprig to garnish

Toasted pitta bread to serve

1. Cut the cucumbers into 5mm dices. Chop the spring onions and garlic very finely
2. Beat the yoghurt in a bowl until smooth, if necessary, the gently stir in the cucumber, spring onions, garlic and mint
3. Add salt and plenty of ground black pepper to taste, then transfer the mixture into a serving bowl. Cover and chill in the refrigerator until ready to serve
4. Garnish with a mint spring and serve with pitta bread

Variations

A similar but smoother dip can be made in the food processor. Peel the mini cucumber and process with two garlic cloves and 3 cups of mixed herbs to a puree. Stir the puree into 1 cup of sour cream and season to taste with salt and pepper.

Cook's tip

Choose Greek-style (US strained plain) yoghurt fir the dip. It has a higher fat content the most yoghurt, which gives the dish a deliciously rich creamy texture.

Recipe #18; Cacik

This refreshing yoghurt dish is served all over the Eastern Mediterranean, whether as part of the mezze with marinated olives and pitta bread or as an accompaniment to meat dishes. Greek tzatziki is very similar serves 6

Ingredients

1 small cucumber

300ml thick natural yoghurt

3 garlic cloves, crushed

2 tbsp chopped fresh mint

2 tbsp chopped fresh dill or parsley

Salt and ground black pepper

Mint or parsley and dill to garnish

Olive oils, olives and pitta bread to serve

1. Finely chop the cucumber and layer in a coriander. Sprinkle with salt to cover the cucumber and position the colander over a bowl to catch the juices that run out. Leave to stand for 30 minutes
2. Wash the cucumber in several changes of cold water to remove the salt and drain it thoroughly. Pat the diced cucumber dry on kitchen paper.
3. Mix together the natural yoghurt, garlic, fresh herbs until the ingredients are thoroughly combined and season with salt and ground black pepper. Stir in the cucumber
4. Garnish with herbs, drizzle over a little olive oil and serve with olives and pitta bread

Cook's tip

The fresh herbs used in this recipe- mint, dill and parsley are simple to grow yourself. Buy a plant of each herb and keep them on a sunny windowsill in your kitchen. Ensure they are kept moist but don't over water them. Pull off the leaves as and when you need them. They will regrow in a matter of days. Keep any mint plants separate from other herbs in their own container as they are very invasive and will rapidly spread

Recipe #19; Lemon and Coconut Dhal Dip

A warm spicy dish, this can be served either as a dip or as an accompaniment to cold meats. Serves 6-8

Ingredients

5cm piece fresh root ginger

1 onion

2 garlic cloves

2 small fresh red chilies, seeded

30ml sunflower oil

5ml cumin seed

150g cup red lentils

250ml cup water

15ml hot curry paste

1 cup coconut cream

Juice of lemon

Handful of fresh coriander leaves

25g flaked almonds

Salt and ground black pepper

1. Use a vegetable peeler to peal the ginger, then cop it finely with the onion, garlic and chilies.
2. Heat the sunflower oil in a large, shallow pan. Add ginger, onions, garlic, chilies and cumin. Cook over a medium heat, stirring occasionally, for about 5 minutes until the onion is softened but not colored
3. Stir the lentils, measured water and curry paste into the pan. Bring to the boil, and then reduce the heat to low. Cover and simmer gently. Stirring occasionally for 15-20 minutes until the lentils are tender but not broken up.
4. Stir in all but 30ml of coconut cream. Bring to the boil and cook, uncovered, for 15-20 minutes, until the mixture is thick and pulpy. Remove the pan from the heat, stir in the lemon juice and coriander leaves. Season to taste
5. Heat a large, heavily pan and dry fry the flaked almonds for about 1-2 minutes on each side, until golden brown. Stir about three quarters of the toasted almonds in the the dhal. Reserve the remainder for the garnish
6. Transfer the dhal to a serving bowl, swirl in the remaining coconut cream. Sprinkle the reserved almonds on top and serve warm.

Chapter 5: Delicious Recipes 1

Recipe #1: Pretzels

These breads are ideal for a buffet or Picnic. Serves 4

Ingredients

For the yeast sponge

10g fresh yeast

5 tbsp water

1 tbsp unbleached plain all purpose white flour

For dough

10g fresh yeast

150ml cup of luke warm water

5 tbsp luke warm milk

3 cups unbleached strong white bread flour

7.5ml salt

2 tbsp butter, melted

For topping

1 egg York

1 tbsp milk

Salt to sprinkle

1. Flour two baking sheets and grease them. Cream the yeast for the yeast sponge with the water. Add the flour, cover and stand at room temperature for 2 hours
2. Mix the yeast for the dough with the water, then stir in the milk, sifts 250g cups of the flour and salt into the bowl. Add the yeast sponge and the butter and mix for 5 minutes. Turn out on to a floured surface and knead in the remaining flour. Place in an oiled bowl, cover with lightly oiled clear film and leave to rise in a warm place for 30 minutes.
3. Turn out on to a floured surface and knock back the dough. Return to the bowl, cover and leave for 30 minutes
4. Turn out the dough onto a floured surface, divide into 12 pieces and form into balls. Roll each ball into a stick. Bend each end into a hoarse hoe. Cross over and place the ends on top of the thick part.
5. Place of the floured and greased baking sheets and let rest for 10 minutes. Preheat the oven to 190c. Bring a large pan of water to the boil, and then simmer the pretzels, in batches for about 1 minute. Drain and place on the greased baking sheets. Mix the egg York and milk and brush over the pretzels. Sprinkle with salt or seeds and bake the pretzels for 25 minutes

Recipe #2: Cheese and Potato Bread Twists

A complete plough man's lunch with the cheese cooked right in the bread. It makes an excellent base for a filling of smoked salmon. Serves 4

Ingredients

250g potatoes, diced

2 cups strong white bread flour

5ml easy blend dried yeast

150ml lukewarm water

2 cups red Leicester cheese, finely grated

2 tbsp olive oil for greasing salt

1. Cook the potatoes in a large pan with plenty of lightly salted boiling water for 20 minutes or until tender. Drain through a colander and return to the pan. Mash until smooth and set aside to cool.
2. Meanwhile sift the flour into a large bowl and add yeast and a good pinch of salt. Stir in the potatoes and rub with your fingers to form a crumb constituency.
3. Make a well in the centre and pour in the water. Start by bringing the mixture together with a round bladed knife, and then use your hands. Knead for several minutes on a well floured surface. Return the dough to the bowl. Cover with a damp cloth and leave to rise in a warm place for 1 hour or until double in size.
4. Turn the dough out and knock back the air bubbles. Knead again for a few seconds. Divide the dough into 12 pieces and shape into rounds
5. Sprinkle the cheese over the baking sheet. Take each ball of dough and roll it in the cheese. Roll each cheese covered roll on a dry surface to long sausages shape. Fold the two ends together and twist the bread. Lay the bread twists on the oiled baking sheet.
6. Cover with a damp cloth and leave the bread to rise in a warm place for 30 minutes. Pre heat the oven to 220c. Bake the bread for 10 to 15 minutes. Serve hot or cold.

Recipe #3: Pepitas

These crunchy spicy and slightly sweet pumpkin seeds are absolutely irresistible, especially if you use hot and tasty chipote chillies to spice then up. Serve bowls of pepitas with pre dinner drinks as an alternative to nuts. Serves 4-6

Ingredients

2 cups pumpkin seeds

8 garlic cloves crushed

Salt

4 tbsp crushed dried chilies

2 tbsp caster sugar

2 wedges of lime

1. Heat a small heavy frying pan; add the pumpkin seeds and dry fry for a few minutes. Stirring constantly as they swell.
2. When all the seeds have swollen, add the garlic and cook for a few more minutes stirring constantly. Add the salt and the crushed chilies and stir to mix. Turn off the heat, but keep the pan on the stove. Sprinkle the sugar over the seeds and shake the pan to make sure that they are all coated
3. Transfer the pepitas into the serving bowl and serve them with the 2 wedges of lime for squeezing over the seeds. If the lime is omitted, the seeds can be cooled and stored in an airtight container for serving cold or reheating later, but they are best served fresh and warm.

Cook's Tip

It's important to keep the pumpkin seeds moving as you cook. Watch them carefully and do not let them burn, or they will taste bitter.

Chipotle chilies are smoke dried jalapeno chilies

Variations

If you are serving the pepitas cold, they can be mixed with cashew nuts and dried cranberries to make a spicy and fruity bowl of nibbles

Recipe #4: Roasted Coconut Cashew Nuts

Serve these sweet and hot cashew nuts at parties. Not only do they taste terrific and look enticing, but the cones help to keep clothes and hands clean and can be thrown away after eating the stuffed contents. These sweet and hot cashew nuts in paper at parties, Serves6-8

Ingredients

1 tbsp ground nut oil

2 tbsp clear honey

2 cups cashew nuts

Cup desiccated dry unsweetened shredded coconut

Small fresh red chilies, seeded and finely chopped

Salt and ground black pepper

7. Heat the oil in the wok or large heavy frying pan and

stir in the honey. After a short while add the coconut and nuts, and stir fry till all sides are golden brown

8. Add the chilies, salt and pepper to taste. Toss until all the ingredients are well mixed. Serve warm or cooled in paper cones or on skewers

Cook's tip

For deep fried cashew nuts, mix 300g cashew nuts with 1 tbsp paprika. 2.5ml turmeric, salt and water in a bowl. Leave the nuts to soak in the spices for an hour. Heat the oil for deep frying in a large pan or wok and fry the nuts until evenly browned. Remove with a slotted spoon and drain on a kitchen towel. Transfer to a serving dish and sprinkle with a little chilli powder

Recipe #5: Spicy Noodle Pancakes

The delicate rice noodle puff up in the hot oil give a fabulous crunchy bite that melts in the mouth. For maximum enjoyment, serve the golden pancakes the moment they are ready and savor the wonderfully crisp texture and the subtle blend of spices. Serve 4

Ingredients

150g dried thin rice noodles

1 fresh red chili, finely diced

2 tbsp finely chopped

2 tsp garlic

1 tsp ground ginger

Small red onion very finely chopped

1 tsp finely chopped lemon grass

1 tsp ground cumin

1 tsp ground coriander

Large pinch of ground turmeric

Salt

Vegetable oil, for frying

Sweet chili sauce for dipping

4. Roughly break up the noodle and place the noodles in a large bowl. Pour over enough boiling water to cover, and soak for about 4-5 minutes. Drain and rinse under cold water. Dry on kitchen towel.
5. Transfer the noodles to a bowl and add the chili, garlic, salt, ground pepper, red onion, lemon grass, ground cumin, coriander and turmeric. Toss well to mix and season with salt.
6. Heat oil in a wok. Working in batches, drop tablespoon of the noodle mixture into the oil. Flatten using the back of a simmer and cook for 2 minutes on each side until crisp and golden. Lift out from the wok.
7. Drain the noodle pancakes on kitchen paper and carefully transfer to a plate or deep bowl. Serve immediately with the chili sauce for dipping.

Cook's tip

For deep frying choose very thin rice noodles. These can be cooked dry but here are soaked and seasoned first.

Chapter 6: Delicious Recipes 2

Recipe #6: Coconut Chips

Coconut chips are a tasty nibble to serve with drinks. The chips can be sliced ahead of time and frozen without salt, on open trays. When frozen, simply shake into plastic boxes. You can then take out as many as you wish for the party.
Serves 8

Ingredients

1 fresh coconut

Salt

7. Preheat the oven to 160c. first drain the coconut juice, either by piercing one of the coconut eyes with a sharp instrument or by breaking it carefully.
8. Lay the coconut on a board and hit the centre sharply with a hammer. The shell should break cleanly in two.
9. Having opened the coconut, use a broad bladed knife to ease the flesh away from the hard outer shell. Taste the piece of the flesh just to make sure it is fresh. Peel away the brown skin with a potato peeler if you like.
10. Slash the coconut flesh into wafer thin shavings, using a food processor, mandolin or sharp knife. Sprinkle the shavings evenly all over one or two baking sheets and sprinkle with salt.
11. Bake for about 30 minutes or until crisp, turning them from time to time. Cool and serve. Any leftover can be stored in airtight containers.

Cook's Tip

This is the kind of recipe where the slicing blade on a food processor comes into its worth preparing two or three coconuts at a time and freezing surplus chips. The chips can be cooked from frozen, but will need to be spread out on the baking sheets, before being salted. Allow a little longer for frozen chips to cook

Recipe #7: Curry Crackers

Crisp curry flavored crackers are very good with creamy cheese or yogurt dips and make an unusual nibble with pre dinner drinks. Add a pinch of cayenne pepper for an extra kick. Serves 6-8

Ingredient
1 cup self rising flour
Pinch of salt
2 tsp garam masala
6 tbs butter, diced
1 tbs finely chopped fresh coriander
1 egg beaten

For topping
Beaten egg
Black onion seeds
Garam masala

5. Preheat the oven to 200c. Put the flour, salt and garam masala into a bowl. Rub in the butter until the mixture resembles fine breadcrumbs. Stir in the coriander, add the egg and mix to a soft dough.
6. Turn out onto a lightly floured surface and knead gently until smooth. Roll out to a thickness of about 3mm.
7. Using a fluted biscuit (cookie) wheel, knife or pizza

wheel, cut the dough into neat rectangles measuring 7cm by 3 cm. Brush with a little beaten egg and sprinkle each cracker with a few black onion seeds. Place on non stick baking sheets and bake in the oven for about 12 minutes until the crackers are light golden brown all over.

8. Remove from oven and transfer onto a wire rack using a metal spatula. Put a little garam masala in a saucer and with a dry pastry brush and dust each cracker with a little of the spice mixture. Leave to cool before serving.

Cook's Tip

Garam masala is a mixture of Indian spices that usually contains a blend of cinnamon, cloves, peppercorns, cardamom seeds and cumin seeds. You can buy it readymade or make your own.

Recipe #8: Sweet and Salty Beetroot Crisps

The Spanish love new and colorful snacks. Try these brightly colored crisps which make an appealing alternative to potato crisps. US potato crisps. Serve them with a bowl of creamy, garlicky mayonnaise and use the crisps to scoop it up. Serves 4

Ingredients

! Small fresh beet root

Caster sugar and fine

Salt for sprinkling

Olive oil for frying

Coarse sea salt to serve

6. Peel the beetroot and using a mandolin or a vegetable peeler, cut into very thin slices
7. Place the beetroot slices on kitchen paper. Spread them out the sprinkle with sugar and fine salt.
8. Put oil into a deep pan to a depth of your desire. Heat it up or until a bread cube added to the hot oil, turns golden brown in 1 minute. Cook the slices in batches until they float to the surface and turn golden brown at the edges. Drain on kitchen paper and sprinkle with sea salt when cool.

Cook's Tip

Don't fry too many beetroot slices at once. They may stick together and not become crisp. If you use a chip basket it will be easy to lift cooked crisps out so they can be drained on kitchen paper. Each batch hot while cooking the remainder.

Variations

Beetroot crisps are particularly flavorsome but other naturally sweet root vegetables such as carrots and sweet potatoes also taste delicious when cooked in this way. You might like to make several different varieties using a mixture of different vegetables and serve them heaped in separate small bowls.

Recipe #9: Peanut Crackers

Theses tasty nutty crackers are ideal as a welcoming appetizer to take the edge off your hunger while you wait for your meal. Serves 4-8

Ingredients

1 cup rice flour

1 tbsp baking powder

1 tsp turmeric powder

1 tbsp ground coriander

1 cup coconut oil

1 cup unsalted peanuts coarsely chopped and crushed

3 candlenuts crushed

3 garlic cloves crushed

Corn or groundnuts peanut oil for shallow frying

Salt and ground black pepper

Chili samabal for dipping (optional)

To season

1 tbsp paprika or fine chili flakes

Salt

6. Put the rice flour, baking powder, ground turmeric and ground coriander into a bowl. Make a well in the centre, pour in the coconut milk and stir well, drawing in the flour from the sides. Beat well to make a smooth batter.
7. Add the peanuts candlenuts and garlic and mix well together. Season with salt and pepper, then put aside for 30 minutes
8. Meanwhile in a small bowl prepare the seasoning by mixing the paprika or fine chili flakes with a little salt.
9. Heat a thin layer of oil in a wok or large frying pan

and drop in a spoonful of batter for each cracker the size of the spoon doesn't matter at the crackers is supposed to vary in size.

10. Work in batches flipping the crackers over when the lacy edges become crispy and golden brown. Drain on kitchen paper and toss them into a basket.
11. Sprinkle the paprika and salt over the crackers and toss them lightly for an even dusting of seasoning
12. Serve the peanut crackers immediately, while they are still warm and crisp. Dip them into some chili sauce if you like.

Recipe #10: Parmesan Thins

These thin crisp savory snacks will melt in the mouth, so make plenty for guest. They are a great treat at any time of the day. So just don't make them for parties and picnics. Serve 8-10

Ingredients

50g plain flour

3 tbsp butter softened

1 egg York

40g freshly grated parmesan cheese

Pinch of salt

Pinch of mustard powder

3. Run together the butter and the flour in a bowl using your hands then work in the egg York.
4. Add the egg York, parmesan and the mustard into the flour mixture. Mix the ingredients thoroughly and

then bring the dough together into a bowl.

5. Shape the dough mixture into a long log wrap the dough long tightly into a plasting film and chill in the refrigerator for 10 minutes.
6. Preheat the oven into 200c. cut the parmesan log into very thin slices and arrange on the baking sheet.
7. Flatted each thin slice with a fork to give a ribbed texture or pattern as you prefer. Bake for about 10 minutes until the crackers are crisp but not changing the color.

Cook's Tip

The quality of parmesan cheese is essential in this recipe. Although parmesan is made in various countries, such as Australia and the USA the best by far is the Italian version called parmigiano reggiano. It may be more expensive than the other varieties but it is well worth the cost.

Chapter 7: Delicious Recipes 3

Recipe #11: Prawn Toasts with Sesame Seeds

This healthy version of the ever popular appetizer has lost none of its classic crunch and taste. Serve it as a snack too. It is great for getting a party off to a good start. Serve 4-6

Ingredients

6 slices medium cut white bread crust removed

225g raw tiger prawns peeled and deveined

50g drained canned water chestnuts

1 egg white

1 tbsp sesame oil

2 tbsp salt

2 spring onions (scallions) finely chopped

2 tbsp dry sherry

1 tbsp sesame seed toasted

Shredded spring onion to garnish

6. Preheat the oven to 200c. cut each slice of bread into four triangles. Spread out on a baking sheet and bake for 25 minutes or until crisp.
7. Meanwhile, put the prawns in a food processor with the water chestnuts, egg, oil and salt. Process the

mixture using the pulse facility until a coarse puree is formed

8. Scrape the mixture into a bowl and stir in the chopped spring onions and sherry and set aside for 10 minutes at room temperature to allow the flavors to blend.

9. Remove the toast from the oven and raise the temperature to 200c. Spread the prawn mixture on the toast. Sprinkle with the sesame seeds and bake for 12 minutes. Garnish the prawn toasts with spring onion and serve hot or warm.

Cook's Tip

Ton toast seeds put them in a dry frying pan and place over medium heat until seeds change color. Shake the pan constantly so the seeds brown evenly and do not burn.

Recipe #12: Spicy Moroccan Olives

Green olives marinated In these two spicy herbal concoctions are simple and quick to prepare and absolutely delicious. Serves 6-8

Ingredients

3 cups green olives for each marinade

3tbsp chopped coriander (cilantro)

3 tbsp chopped fresh flat leaf of parsley

1 garlic clove finely chopped

Good pinch of cayenne pepper

Good pinch of ground cumin

3 tbsp olive oil plus extra if necessary

3 tbsp lemon juice plus extra if necessary

For the hot chili marinade

4 tbsp chopped fresh coriander

4tbsp fresh chopped flat leaf of parsley

I garlic clove finely chopped

1 tbsp finely grated ginger root

1 red chili seeded ad diced

1 preserved lemon cut into stripes

5. Crack the olives hard enough to break the flesh but taking care not to crack the pits. Place in a bowl of cold water and leave over night to remove the excess brine. Drain thoroughly and divide the olives between two jars.
6. Mix all the ingredients for the spicy herbal marinade in a jug. Pour over the olives in adding more olive and lemon juice to cover if necessary.
7. To make the hot chili marinade, mix all the ingredients. Pour over the olives in the second jar. Store both the jars in the refrigerator for at least 1 week shaking the occasionally.

Variations

A jar of marinated olives makes a perfect present for anyone who appreciates their flavor. Experiment with herbs and spices in the marinade, try oregano and basil and substitute lime juice for the lemon juice or even use flavored vinegars

Recipe #13: Tapas of Almonds, Olive and Cheese.

Serving a few choice nibbles with drinks is the perfect way to get an evening off to a good start and when you can get everything ready ahead of time life's easier round. Serve 6-8

Ingredients

For marinated Olives

2.5ml coriander seeds

2.5ml fennel seeds

2 garlic cloves crushed

1 tbsp chopped fresh rosemary

10ml chopped fresh parsley

1 tbsp vinegar

2 tbsp olive oil

115g black olives

115g green olives

For the marinated cheese

150g manchego or other firm cheese

6 tbsp olive oil

1 tbsp white wine vinegar

1 tbsp black peppercorns

1 garlic clove sliced

Fresh thyme or tarragon springs

Fresh flat leaf of parsley or tarragon

Sprigs to garnish

For the salted almonds

1.5ml cayenne pepper

2 tbsp sea salt

2 tbsp butter

4 tbsp olive oil

1 cup blanked almonds

5. To make the marinated olives crush the coriander and fennel seeds in a mortar with pestle. Work in the garlic, and then add the rosemary, parsley, vinegar and olive oil. Mix well. Put the olives in a small bowl and pour the marinated. Cover with clear film (plastic wrap) and chill for up to 1 week.

6. To make the marinated cheese, cut the manchego or other firm cheese into bite size pieces, removing any rind and put in a small bowl. Combine the oil. Vinegar, peppercorns, garlic, thyme or tarragon and pour over the cheese. Cover with clear film and chill for up to 3 days.

7. To make the salted almonds, combine the cayenne

pepper and salt in a bowl. Melt the butter with the oil in a frying pan. Add the almonds in to the salt mixture and toss until they are evenly coated. Leave to cool then store upto 1 week. Serve the almonds olives and cheese in separate dishes.

Recipe #14: Tapenade and Aioli with Vegetables

These summer vegetables with tapenade and aioli make an excellent appetizer. Serve 6

Ingredients

1 cup pitted black olives

2oz can anchovy fillets drained

Half a cup olive oil

Finely grated rind of 1 lemon

1 tbsp brandy (optional)

Ground black pepper

For the herb aioli

2 egg yolks

1 tbsp dijan mustard

2 tbsp white wine vinegar

250ml light olive oil

3 tbsp chopped mixed fresh herbs such as chervil

Parsley

2tbsp chopped watercress

5 garlic cloves crushed

Salt and ground black pepper

225g asparagus young

12 quail's eggs

Fresh herbs to garnish

Coarse salt for sprinkling

7. Make the tapenade. Finely chop the olives, anchovies
    and capers and beat with the oil and lemon rind and
    brandy, if using any.
8. To make the aioli, beat together the egg yolks,
    mustard and vinegar. Whisk in the oil a trickle at a
    time, until it gets thick and smooth. Season and add
    the herbs, watercress and garlic. Cover and chill.
9. Put the peppers on a foil lined grill rack and brush
    with oil. Cook under high heat until just beginning to
    char.
10. Cook the potatoes in boiling water until tender. Add
    the beans and carrots and cook for 1 minute. Add the
    asparagus and cook for another 30 seconds. Drain the
    vegetables.
11. Cook the quail eggs in boiling water for 2 minutes.
    Drain and remove half of each shell. Arrange all the
    vegetables, eggs and sauces on the serving platter.
    Garnish with fresh herbs and serve with coarse salt for
    sprinkling.

Recipe #15: Olive and Anchovy Bites

These little melt in the mouth morsels are very moreish and are perfect accompaniment for drinks. They are made from two ingredients that are forever associated with tapas and are included in many traditional recipes. Olives and anchovies. The reason for this is that both contain plenty of salt which helps to stimulate thirst and therefore drinking. Makes 40-50

Ingredients

1 cup plain flour

115g chilled butter diced

1 cup finely chopped manchego mature (sharp)

Cheddar or gruyere cheese

50g can anchovy fillets in oil

Drained and roughly chopped

1 cup pitted black olives roughly chopped

2.5ml cayenne pepper sea salt to serve.

1. Place the flour, butter, cheese, anchovies, olives and cayenne pepper in a food processor and process into a firm dough.
2. Wrap the dough loosely into a clear film (plastic wrap) chill for 20 minutes
3. Pre heat the oven into 200c. roll out the dough thinly on a lightly floured surface.
4. Cut the dough into 5cm wide stripes, then cut across each strip in alternative directions to make triangles. Transfer to baking sheet and bake for 8 – 10 minutes

until golden. Cool on a wire rack. Sprinkle with sea salt before serving.

Variations

To add a little extra spice, dust the olive and anchovy bites lightly with cayenne pepper before baking.

Crisp little nibbles set off most drinks. Serve this nibbles bites alongside a little bowl of seeds and nuts such as sunflower seeds and pistachios. These come in the shell, the opening of which provides a diversion while chatting and gossiping. Toasted chickpeas are another popular tapas snack.

Chapter 8: Delicious Recipe 4

Recipe #16: Anchovy and Caper Bites

These miniature skewers are very popular in Spain, where they are called pinchos which literally means stuck on a thorn. Taste color and shape guide the choice of ingredients that are speared together on cocktail sticks. The selection may also include pieces of cold or salted fish or even hard boiled edges. In the south of the country piquant pickled vegetables are the most popular combination. In that region, the resemblance of the little sticks to a bullfighters dart was noticed and so the dish was reamed pinchos. Serves 4.

Ingredients

12 small capers

12 canned anchovy fillets in oil, drained

12 pitted black olives

12 cornichons or small gherkins

12 silverskin pickled onions

1. Using your finger, place a caper are the thicker end of each anchovy fillet and carefully roll it up so that the caper is completely enclosed
2. Thread the caper filled anchovy, one olive, one cornichon or gherkin and one pickled onion on to each other of 12 cocktail sticks (toothpicks). Chill and serve.

Cook's Tip

If the anchovies you are suing are extremely salty, try soaking them in a little milk before using them. Salted caper should also be rinsed before use.

Variations

Add a chunk of canned tuna in oil to each stick. You can vary the ingredients if you like, using slices of cold meats, chunks of cheese and pickled vegetable. Choose a selection of three or four ingredients to give contrasting textures flavors and colors.

Recipe #17: Crap Egg rolls

These appetizers are similar to Chinese spring rolls and ideal for buffets, parties and summer picnics. Serve 6-8

Ingredients

3 eggs

1 cup plain flour sifted

2.5ml salt

Vegetable oil for deep frying

3 tbsp light soy sauce mixed with 1 tbsp sesame oil for dipping

Lime wedges to serve

For fillings

225g white crab meat or small prawns(shrimp)

3 large spring onions (scallion) shredded

1 piece fresh root ginger diced

2 garlic cloves crushed

1 tbsp soy sauce

2-3 tbsp corn flour blended with water

1 egg separated

Salt and ground pepper

1. Lightly beat the eggs and gradually stir in the water. Put the flour and salt into another bowl and work in the egg in the mixture. Blend to a smooth batter, then leave to rest for 20 minutes.
2. Grease a 25cm frying pan and heat gently. Whisk the batter then pour then pour into the pan and spread it very thinly. Cook for 2 minutes or until set underneath. There is no need to cook the pancakes on the other side. Make further 11 pancakes cooked side upwards between sheets of baking parchment. Set aside until ready to use.
3. To make the fillings combine the crab and prawns, spring onions, ginger, garlic, bamboo shoots or bean sprouts, soy sauce, corn flour and water, egg yolk and seasoning. Lightly beat the egg white. Place a spoonful of filling in the middle of each pancake, brush the edges with egg white and fold into parcels tucking in the ends.
4. Heat the oil in a heavy frying pan. When the cube of bread turns brown after dropping it in the hot oil in one minute, carefully add the four parcels. Cook for 2 minutes or until golden brown. Remove and place on kitchen towel to drain the extra oil and cook the remaking egg rolls. Serve with the soy sauce dip and

sesame oil dip and wedges of lemon or lime.

Recipe #18: Shiitake and Scallop Bundles

A wok does double duty for making these delicate mushroom and sea food treats, first for steaming and then for deep frying. Serves 4.

Ingredients

4 scallops

8 large fresh shiitake mush rooms

225g long yam unpeeled

4tbsp miso

1 cup fresh breadcrumbs

Corn flour for dusting

Vegetable oil for deep frying

Salt

4 lemon wedges to serve

1. Slice the scallops in two into horizontally, and then sprinkle with salt. Remove the stalks from the shiitake and discard them. Cut shallow slits on the top of the shiitake to form a hash symbol. Sprinkle with a little salt.
2. Heat the steamer and steam the long yam for 10 to 15 minutes or until soft. Test with a skewer; remove to cool the remove the skin. Mash the flesh in the bowl add the miso the mix well.

3. Take the bread crumbs in in your hands then break them finely. Mix the half into the mashed long yam and set aside the rest on a side plate.

4. Fill the underneath of the shiitake caps with a scoop of the mashed long yam. Smooth down with the flat edge of a knife and dust the mash with corn flour. Add a little mash to a slice of scallop and place on top.

5. Spread another mashed long yam onto of a scallop and shape to completely cover. Make sure that all the ingredients are clinging together. Repeat to make 8 little mounds.

6. Place the beated egg in a shallow container. Dust the shiitake and the scallop mounds with corn flour, and then dip into the egg. Handle with care as the scallops and mashed yams are quite soft. Coat well with the bread crumbs and fry in the hot oil until golden brown. Drain well on kitchen pepper. Serve hot on individual plates with a wedge of fresh cut lemon.

Recipe #19: Thai Fish Cakes with Cucumber Relish

These wonderful little nibbles are very familiar and popular appetizers. Serves 4

Ingredients

300g white fish fillet such as cod cut into cubes

2 tbsp Thai fish sauce

1 egg

2 tbsp corn flour

3 kaffr lime leaves shredded

1 tbsp chopped fresh coriander (cilantro)

50g green beans thinly sliced

Vegetable oil for frying

Chinese mustard cress to garnish

For cucumber relish

4 tbsp rice vinegar

4 tbsp water

50g cup sugar

1 cucumber, quartered and sliced

4 shallots thinly sliced

1 tbsp chopped fresh root ginger

1. To make the cucumber relish brings the vinegar, water and sugar to the boil. Stir until the sugar dissolves the remove from the heat and leave to cool.
2. Combine the rest of the relish ingredients together in a bowl and pour the vinegar mixture over.
3. Combine the fish, curry paste and egg in a food processor and process until combined. Transfer the mixture into a bowl, add the Thai fish sauce, sugar, corn flour, lime leaves, coriander and green beans and mix well.
4. Mould and shape the mixture into patties about 5cm in diameter and 5mm in thickness.
5. Heat the oil in a wok or deep fryer. Add the fish cakes in small batches and deep fry for about 4 to 5 minutes or until golden brown. Remove and drain well on a kitchen paper. Keep the cooked fish cakes arm in a low oven while you cook the remainder. Garnish with

Chinese mustard cress and serve immediately with a little cucumber spooned on the side.

Conclusion

Thank you again for purchasing this book on *Delicious Appetizers*.

I am extremely excited to pass this information along to you, and I am so happy that you now have read and can hopefully implement these strategies going forward.

I hope this book was able to help you understand the basic idea of eating well and living a healthy life.

The next step is to get started using this information and to hopefully live a healthier yet frugal life! Please don't be someone who just reads this information and doesn't apply it, the strategies in this book will only benefit you if you use them!

If you know of anyone else that could benefit from the information presented here please inform them of this book.

Finally, if you enjoyed this book and feel it has added value to your life in any way, please take the time to share your thoughts and post a review on Amazon. It'd be greatly appreciated!

Thank you and good luck!

Legal Notice

Disclaimer Notice